KETOGENIC MEAL PREP

Beginners Guide to Meal Prep 4-Weeks of Ketogenic Diet Recipes (28 Full Days of Keto Meals)

Olivia Rogers

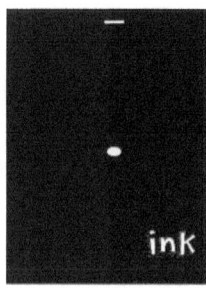

First published in 2019 by Venture Ink Publishing

Copyright © The Menu At Home 2019

All rights reserved.

No part of this book may be reproduced in any form without permission in writing from the author. No part of this publication may be reproduced or transmitted in any form or by any means, mechanic, electronic, photocopying, recording, by any storage or retrieval system, or transmitted by email without the permission in writing from the author and publisher.

Requests to the publisher for permission should be addressed to publishing@ventureink.co

For more information about the contents of this book or questions to the author, please contact Olivia Rogers at olivia@themenuathome.com

Disclaimer

This book provides wellness management information in an informative and educational manner only, with information that is general in nature and that is not specific to you, the reader. The contents of this book are intended to assist you and other readers in your personal wellness efforts. Consult your physician regarding the applicability of any information provided in this book to you.

Nothing in this book should be construed as personal advice or diagnosis, and must not be used in this manner. The information provided about conditions is general in nature. This information does not cover all possible uses, actions, precautions, side-effects, or interactions of medicines, or medical procedures. The information in this book should not be considered as complete and does not cover all diseases, ailments, physical conditions, or their treatment.

You should consult with your physician before beginning any exercise, weight loss, or health care program. This book should not be used in place of a call or visit to a competent health-care professional. You should consult a health care professional before adopting any of the suggestions in this book or before drawing inferences from it.

Any decision regarding treatment and medication for your condition should be made with the advice and consultation of a qualified health care professional. If you have, or suspect you have, a health-care problem, then you should immediately contact a qualified health care professional for treatment.

No Warranties: The author and publisher don't guarantee or warrant the quality, accuracy, completeness, timeliness, appropriateness or suitability of the information in this book, or of any product or services referenced in this book.

The information in this book is provided on an "as is" basis and the author and publisher make no representations or warranties of any kind with respect to this information. This book may contain inaccuracies, typographical errors, or other errors.

Liability Disclaimer: The publisher, author, and other parties involved in the creation, production, provision of information, or delivery of this book specifically disclaim any responsibility, and shall not be held liable for any damages, claims, injuries, losses, liabilities, costs, or obligations including any direct, indirect, special, incidental, or consequences damages (collectively known as "Damages") whatsoever and howsoever caused, arising out of, or in connection with the use or misuse of the site and the information contained within it, whether such Damages arise in contract, tort, negligence, equity, statute law, or by way of other legal theory.

Table of Contents

Disclaimer	3
Who Is This Book For?	7
What Will This Book Teach You?	9
Introduction	11
Chapter 1: How Does The Keto Diet Work	13
Chapter 2: Meal Prepping For Beginners	29
Chapter 3: Keto Meal Prep	42
Conclusion	112
Final Words	114

Who Is This Book For?

If you want to get on an efficient diet plan that doesn't involve anything as bothersome as counting calories, or as drastic as severely reducing your portion sizes, but you don't know where to start; congratulations! This book is for you.

With so many fads going on, especially regarding diets, trusting any kind of health practice is not an easy proposition. This book is here to help you remove the shroud.

Many trending diets come and go, followed by an expected scarcity of long-term success. Most of those are based on novelty concepts that are miles away from science and reproducibility.

This book is directed towards the concerned person, looking to get down to the nitty-gritty of eating healthily. However, it will provide much more than that, and even the more inquisitive readers will get to satisfy their curiosity about the nutritional processes involved!

What Will This Book Teach You?

In this book, you will learn all about the Keto diet: how does it work, why you should consider it, what boons will it bring to your life, what details you must consider, and what is the best way to complement it.

Each and every explanation made will be delivered along with facts; understanding Keto entails unlearning some wrong practices we've been taught our entire lives.

Besides this, you will go over the concept of proper meal preparation, henceforth referred to as meal prep, and its many benefits. You'd be surprised to know just how much control and freedom you can get out of planning your meals in time.

Armed with this knowledge, you will be given 4-weeks' worth of Keto meal prep, which will include breakfast, lunch, dinner, and, of course, snacks!

The goal is providing the reader with the knowledge to eat healthily and in accordance to the Keto diet, while enjoying tasty food and snacks! A diet *does not* have to be boring or dull to be effective after all.

Introduction

The "Keto" diet—more precisely, the ketogenic diet—is an extraordinarily low-carb dietary plan. It contrasts the majority of diets by being high-fat and adequate-protein instead.

It originated in the 1920s, and it was developed by a team of researchers working at Johns Hopkins Hospital to treat patients of refractory epilepsy.

The diet was tremendously effective at improving the condition of those suffering from seizures, especially children, although it has been abandoned now for anticonvulsant drugs, and relegated to being an alternative in the case that patients don't achieve control over their epilepsy.

You might be wondering what does all this have to do with us if we don't suffer from epilepsy. Well, continue reading!

The researchers who developed the diet discovered that fasting could suppress the number of seizure patients suffered while conveying other benefits such as regulated body fat, blood sugar, cholesterol, and hunger.

Now, fasting is obviously not a feasible long-term prospect, so the researchers set about developing a diet to reproduce the beneficial effects of fasting: the ketogenic diet.

The Keto diet tricks the body into thinking it is fasting, bringing forth the associated effects without the real fast. To achieve this, one must conduct a throughout elimination of glucose that is found in carbohydrate foods. Maybe you've heard about a "no-carb" or "low-carb" diet—very likely, those were ketogenic diets.

It basically emulates fasting, but without actually starving your body from necessary calories; you starve your body of carbohydrates.

In the following chapter, we're going to cover all you need to know about the Keto diet before getting down to your meals!

Chapter 1

How Does The Keto Diet Work

The Keto diet severely restricts the intake of almost all foods with sugar and starch; more specifically, carbohydrates in general.

The way these foods are processed is simple: they're broken down into our blood as insulin and glucose, commonly referred to as blood sugar.

This is something completely natural and also necessary for the body. However, when blood sugar's levels go out of control, the extra calories are stored as body fat, resulting in unwanted (and unhealthy) weight gain.

In contrast to this, the Keto diet cuts off the glucose levels due to the low-carb (or even no-carb) dieting, therefore the body is forced to burn fat and produces ketones, which can be measured as well.

Most of us live on a high-carb diet, so our bodies run on glucose for energy as usual. The trick of the diet relies on the fact that our bodies cannot produce glucose on their own; we have barely a day's worth of it stored in our muscle tissue and liver.

At this point, you can see how the Keto diet emulates fasting— Once our body runs out of glucose, and if we don't feed it any from a food source, it be will begin to burn stored fat instead. With the Keto diet, we feed our body enough fat (and get rid of the carbohydrates) to essentially switch from a "Sugar-burner" into a "Fat-burner."

The process inevitably sounds a lot easier than counting calories, actually fasting, or burning loads of calories through a series of explosive and intensive workouts.

Despite the previously mentioned, don't assume that just because you're on a Ketogenic diet you must eat *all* kinds of fats; the Keto diet emphasizes *healthy* fats and less proteins overall, so don't go guzzling bacon!

Ketosis And The Keto Diet

You might be wondering where does the name come from: It comes from Ketosis, a process that takes the reins once the glucose of your body is dramatically reduced—The one we previously described.

Ketosis boosts the production of ketones, which quickly populate your blood until reaching a certain point. Once this state is reached, you enter ketosis: quick and consistent weight loss in favor of a stable body weight.

This is a very complex process of the human body, but we're going to keep it straight-forward. Ketosis occurs the moment your liver starts breaking fat into fatty acids and glycerol, then, your body breaks the fatty acids into ketones, an energy-rich substance, and circulates it through your bloodstream.

Amongst the ketones, you can find three primary types: acetone, beta-hydroxybutyrate, and acetoacetate. The second provides the most energy to the brain, while the latter supplies the most energy to the body.

Going from "sugar-burner" to "fat-burner" is not without its impact—Both physically and mentally, you will feel the difference between being on ketosis and being on glycolysis ("sugar burner").

The general feeling is that ketosis is a "cleaner" way to stay fueled, compared to its alternative. However, it is known as a fact that ketosis *actively* reduces your body weight, while glycolysis can do the opposite.

The Pros Of The Keto Diet

We've covered the main benefit of the ketogenic diet which is the steady, healthy weight loss but there are other benefits to the diet than this!

Reduced Risks For Type 2 Diabetes

The Keto diet reduces the risks for Type 2 diabetes, thanks to its control of insulin release.

When you eat carbohydrates, insulin is released as a response to the elevated blood sugar. The ketogenic diet eliminates carbohydrates from your consumption, preventing the release of inordinate quantities of insulin.

At the same time, it can reverse cases of insulin resistance—current diabetics on insulin should contact their doctor prior to starting the Keto diet though, as insulin dosages might need to be revised.

Cancer Killer

Cancer cells often proliferate on highly-processed, low-nutrient diets. It would require a huge categorical shift in cancer cells so that they could metabolically process fat as well as glucose, if at all.

Due to this, and some studies conducted under this premise, researchers have found some evidence to sustain that a ketogenic diet might be capable of "starving" cancer cells—preventing their development, or even destroying them.

Cholesterol And Blood Pressure Regulator

The Keto diet, despite being high in fat, is unlikely to negatively affect your cholesterol levels.

In some cases, when the patient adheres to the diet for a long period, usually 24 weeks, it can significantly reduce the levels of triglycerides and LDL cholesterol blood; HDL cholesterol levels, however, are boosted. These elements, combined with the natural weight loss of the Keto diet, lean towards normalized blood pressure, which is often related to overweight and obesity.

Neurological Support

The Keto diet has been used to successfully treat and reverse neurological disorders and cognitive impairments for almost a century. Formerly, researchers and medics had assumed that its only use was aiding those suffering from refractory epilepsy and, in some cases, Alzheimer's symptoms.

Nonetheless, such assumptions have been questioned recently, as more and more studies are linking the ketogenic diet with the correction of certain anomalies in cellular energy usage—a characteristic that plagues those who suffer neurological disorders.

The ketogenic diet is capable of enhancing the biogenesis of mitochondria, which at the same time boosts the capacity of brain cells, shielding them from neurodegenerative diseases.

All in all, Keto could be used as a reliable way to reverse and prevent the effects from some of these conditions, especially if the diet is sustained for a long period.

Ketosis For The Brain, Ketones For The Head

Due to the way our bodies burn ketones, a stream of benefits flows right into our brains. For starters, ketones are naturally neuroprotective antioxidants, meaning that they can protect your brain from harmful reactive oxygen species that damage brain cells.

Many of the neurological-related benefits from the Keto diet stem from the way the brain handles its fuel—ketones are more efficient *per unit* than glucose; as the brain ages, its ability to burn fuel deteriorates, meaning that the efficiency of each unit becomes more important.

Lastly, but certainly stellar, ketones are capable of triggering the expression of the Brain-derived neurotrophic factor (BDNF for short) which is responsible for the support, growth, and differentiation of existing and new neurons and neuronal connections.

Such trigger can not only support but *improve* the functions of some brain areas such as the hippocampus, cortex, and basal forebrain—essential parts in the learning, memory, and abstract thinking processes.

Reduced Mortality

A high-carb intake is associated with higher risks of total mortality, unlike total fat which is related to lower total mortality.

A low-carb, high-fat diet is bound to help you live both longer and healthy. In several instances, a saturated fat intake is inversely associated with the risk for suffering a stroke.

Reduced Inflammation

High-carb diets are more often than not pro- inflammatory, and that is usually terrible for your skin.

Switching to a low-carb diet, such as Keto, can successfully reduce the number of lesions and skin inflammations—on the other hand, a high-carb diet does the opposite, and Acne is often linked to high-carb intake.

Those suffering heavy acne might need more than a dietary switch, but for the most cases, a reduced dairy intake and a low-carb diet should get rid of the condition completely.

The Cons Of The Ketogenic Diet

The Keto diet is, however, not without its side-effects. These symptoms stem from the initial metabolic shift, so they should subside in a week or two. The adverse symptoms include:

- Headache
- Bad breath
- Fatigue
- Muscle weakness
- Poor sleep
- Constipation
- Nausea
- Moodiness
- Brain Fog
- No Libido

Adding bone broth to your Keto diet helps restore your electrolytes—It is advised that you drink a lot of water in this diet, but you will nonetheless lose a lot of water weight, and even flush out some essential electrolytes. Bone broth can replenish these naturally, as well as providing you with nutrients and amino acids.

Other foods to consider are nuts, avocados, mushrooms, and other fish. They're particularly good at replenishing your electrolyte intake. You might experience more hunger than usual, in that case it is advised to consume more fat; if low on energy, reduce exercise temporarily.

Lastly, try to ingest low-carb foods that are easy to digest, and don't push the no-carb version of the diet if you're prone to fatigue and weakness when low on carbohydrates.

Keto Diet and Women

Most studies of the ketogenic diet have been conducted using men or animals, not so much for women. It's only natural that its efficiency with women is objected and questioned.

Women's hormones are more sensitive towards dietary and lifestyle changes, but that doesn't mean we can't partake in the Keto diet!

The best advice for any women taking the ketogenic diet is focusing on an alkaline low-carb Keto diet. This alkaline variation of the ketogenic diet can singlehandedly single out the cons of the Keto diet, and it's just as effective on women as it is on men.

Restoring The Alkalinity

Restoring the alkalinity of your body will bring forth other benefits as well, so do try to incorporate some of these alkaline-oriented practices for your low-carb Keto diet if you're dealing with the side-effects of the ketogenic diet:

- Some of the foods you can consider for your alkaline Keto diet are: beet greens, dandelions, spinach, wheat and alfalfa grass, mushrooms, tomatoes, avocado, broccoli, garlic, oregano, radishes, beans, cabbage, and sea veggies.

- Much of your produce is best if eaten raw, or steamed, and you should do it almost all the time if you can.

- Healthy fats are incredibly good for you! Coconut oil, MCT oil, olive oil, grass-fed beef, nuts, wild-caught fish and especially salmon.

- Drink a lot of water, and when you can, drink alkaline water.

- Cut or eliminate the consumption of all sources of (added) sugar, gains, dairy (though very small amounts every now and then can't hurt you, especially cheese), caffeine, alcohol, processed meats, and generally anything that contains a lot of sugar, sodium, fillers, or other synthetic ingredients.

- Get the necessary rest! I can't stress this enough. You should get between 7 and 9 hours of sleep each night.

The Keys Of The Keto Diet

First, you must cut down your glucose consumption: grains, starchy vegetables, fruits, etc. Their consumption *must* be reduced or eliminated.

This will force your body to find an alternative source of fuel: fat. Foods such as avocados, coconut oil, and salmon are very good choices.

Once the body starts burning fat to produce ketones, your blood's ketone levels will rise until you reach ketosis. During this state, you reap the benefits of the Keto diet: fat burn and weight loss.

To attain and maintain ketosis you must change your diet, so you're probably wondering how many carb foods you can eat while being in ketosis.

The most precise answer I can give you is: depends!

You can follow the "traditional" Keto diet which was aimed towards those suffering from epilepsy: 75% of calories from fat sources (think oils and fattier cuts of meat), 5% from carbohydrates, and the remaining 20% from protein.

However, you're not obliged to follow such diet. Instead, you can follow a less-restricting Keto diet which can help you just as well in a safer and reasonably fast way.

The transition must be smooth, as it can convey some side-effects. Broadly speaking, **about 30 to 50 net grams of total carbs daily is good enough to start with.**

Whenever you feel comfortable in this new way of eating, you can lower your carbs even further, to about 20 grams per day (you could to it sporadically from time to time).

The previous approach is what most Keto dieters strive for, as adhering to it will net the best results, but don't forget each person is different, and so is their metabolism.

The rule of thumb here is don't do it if it negatively affects you; you're doing this to enhance your wellbeing, not the contrary.

Stages Of Ketosis

Not formal *per se*, but this segment should give you a realistic expectation, as well as some sort of list you can check to see your progress.

The most difficult part of *all* diets is the beginning, and trust me, it is even more intense for Keto.

The ketogenic diet involves shifting your metabolism in a pretty significant and concise way—For this reason, you must make your transition as smooth and slow as possible; don't be afraid to extend the process beyond what you thought.

Early Stage

As soon as you trigger ketosis, you will inevitably experience some signs and symptoms of your body change. They're colloquially known as the "Keto flu." You will experience some of the side-effects previously covered, and they can dissipate rather quickly, in one to two weeks, but in some cases, they subside after more weeks.

You will likely experience:

- Increased cravings, especially for sugar or carbohydrates. Expected, but you *cannot* give in.

- Constipation.

- Moodiness.

- Lack of energy, bad sleep, and more lasting exertion.

- Loss of libido.

- Bad breath.

The effects should be pretty mild, if apparent at all.

Middle Stage

As your body becomes accustomed to being in ketosis, negative symptoms recede. In turn, you will notice some improvements in your health.

It is important you're able to objectively note them, as they're signs of whether or not you're effectively transitioning into ketosis:

- Less appetite than before, especially if you were prone to overeating.

- Reduced hunger and cravings. Generally, you will feel less desire to eat, only when you feel hungry.

- Increased physical and mental performance, not necessarily an improvement over actual capacity, but rather more sustained energy.

- Progressive weight loss—This one is pretty evident.

Final Stage

Once all side-effects have gone away, you can consider yourself in the final stage. At this point onwards, you must maintain your diet, and especially your blood's ketone levels.

Reverting to glycolysis is completely possible, and doing so won't only render your efforts in vain, but will produce side-effects similar to the ones you experimented in the early stage!

There are many ways of measuring your ketone levels, such as using a blood ketone meter, which is the most precise but also the most expensive; performing urine strip tests, which are cheaper and precise enough (they do not reveal your beta-hydroxybutyrate levels, though); and lastly, you can use a breath analyzer, but they aren't very precise.

Your blood's ketone level is called serum ketone levels, and its value falls between 0.5 to 3.0 mmol/L. "Optimal ketosis" is often considered to be attained with values between 1.5 and 3.

To resume

Ketosis is what keeps our bodies running once the glucose is spent, as we described earlier. However, the brain cannot make use of fats for fuel: that's when ketones step in. Due to our brain's need for fast-acting energy sources, and especially an energy source that doesn't generate too many reactive oxygen species, our liver converts fatty acids into ketones for the brain.

As you know, starving (or prolonged fasting) leads to the accelerated loss of muscle mass in order to keep the fort—your body—standing. Your brain alone would demand over 2 pounds *per day* of lean mass to run; ketones cut the necessary mass loss by fivefold, even more with sufficient protein consumption.

The goal of the ketogenic diet is achieving the ketosis state, without actually starving, in order to fuel your body off the circulation of ketones in your bloodstream. In other words, the goal is *altering* your metabolism.

Such a metabolic change will shift the mechanics you were accustomed to: no longer will your body promote the storage of body fat, nor block its release from adipose tissues, instead, your body will readily release and consume your fat reserves.

The transition must be smooth, you shouldn't *drastically* reduce your carb consumption, let alone eliminate it entirely in one go, as that might amplify the potential side-effects. I recommend you reduce your carb consumption slowly and steadily; let the change sink in for about two to three weeks to avoid complications.

In the following chapter, you will learn more about what you *can* eat, and what you *cannot*. I will also give you a brief introduction to the world of meal prepping—Not only it is more efficient than preparing meal after meal *every* day, it is also the way to go when dieting, as it allows you to avoid excesses, cravings, or mistakes.

Don't be afraid of the Keto diet, there are still plenty tasty things to enjoy, and depending on what you like, you might even prefer the Keto diet for its recipes!

Chapter 2

Meal Prepping For Beginners

The name does sound a bit technical or specific, but in reality, "meal prep" simply refers to the weekly preparation of your meals, covering periods longer than two to three days, often prepared for an entire week.

The meal prep approach is filled with several advantages, such as:

- Time Saving. Preparing a week's worth of meals in advance *will* take a couple of hours. But, think about it! All that time you're spending *in a single day* won't be wasted during the week. Meal prep is bound to cut time spent cooking and preparing food by at least fivefold!

- Money Saving. If you're eating outside, not only you're eating unhealthily most of the time, you're also spending much more money! Just think about how much would you spend per week if you ate lunch and dinner outside every day, compared to preparing your own meals.

- Diet Discipline. When you prepare your meals and snacks in advance, you conform them to your needs and goals; no more mindlessly falling for the cravings or conveniences, your healthy food will be awaiting you!

You might think doing so eliminates variety, takes more time than what it saves, or is actually unhealthy. For each concern you have, I've got something to say!

First, you're only sacrificing variety if you choose to: you're the one who picks the meals you prepare, so everything is on your hands! Worry not, however, this book will offer you thoroughly varied Keto meal prep planning!

Initially, you might spend a lot of time preparing your ingredients, cooking your food, properly storing it, and cleaning up.

Nonetheless, meal prep is a skill, like any other, so it becomes easier as you become experienced. Besides, you can always split your meal prep into two days, rather than one, but you should try to get it all done within a day in order to maximize the time gains!

Lastly, some are concerned with the quality of the food. Broadly speaking, the quality *will* depend on several factors that you can control, such as the quality of your ingredients and storage, as well as the nature of the dishes you wish to prepare. Again, proper meal prep planning solves these issues!

Getting Started

Alright, this should be fairly easy! Before doing your meal prep, pick a day of the week—People often go for Sundays, as they're the day you're off work, and the family is at home, meaning you can get some help from the entire family!

Depending on your life and your schedule, you might wish to split your meal prep in two days, be it for convenience or time. In that case, Wednesday is often a good day after Sunday.

You *must* be disciplined with the day; whether you desire to do your meal prep on Sundays, or on any combination of days, you must *honestly* commit to it—doing so isn't only necessary for the venture to be successful, it will enhance your sense of self-discipline which is perfect for both your diet and your life as a whole!

You might want to limit yourself for just a few meals for a couple of days, in place of an entire week's worth of meals—I actually advise you to prepare for the week, as the process isn't really difficult, and the first experience will give you a proper taste of what is to come. However, do whatever makes you feel comfortable! Each person has their own schedules and preferences.

Note: During this process, it is assumed you're going to prepare the Keto meals for yourself, but you might choose to prepare Keto meals for your family as well—You can always do your own Keto meals and *then* your family's meal, but that will take more time so either clear these details up, or get some help from the household!

Tools And Stock Of The Trade

You won't need anything fancy for your meal prep, well, unless you really want to get technical about it.

Be sure you have the following in your kitchen before heading into the fray:

- A Skillet: Preferably a cast iron one; having extra sizes might be handy, but you need at least one.

- A Chef Knife: The higher the quality, the better. You'll want something sharp, with a stable grip, and a durable edge.

- A food processor: Or a good old blender. Saves a lot of time, and allows you to prepare certain dishes. You might want to have both a blender and a processor though. It's up to you!

- A crockpot: I prefer calling it slow cooker. They're perfect for multitasking, as you can drop and forget your foods there while they cook and you perform other tasks.

- A supply of parchment paper: Prevents sticking when baking, allowing you to do as many divisions in the oven as you want without worrying. They're also super cheap.

With these tools, you're more than ready to commence!

Should you want more finery in your kitchen, there are extra tools you can consider such as a vegetable spiralizer, an immersion blender, a precise kitchen scale, a collection of measuring cups, and the list goes on and on—Most of them are beyond the scope of the book, as they require more cooking expertise than beginner-level Keto meals.

Regarding pantry and general stocking, you should have a few of the following:

- Nuts (and nut butters) and seeds.

- Coconut and almond flour.

- Baking soda and powder, MCT oil powder, and cocoa powder.

- Avocado and coconut oil.

- Yellow mustard (Dijon mustard is good), vanilla extracts, red wine vinegar.

- Salt, pepper, oregano, garlic, parsley, thyme, cinnamon. Celery salt and red pepper flakes are good too.

It is important to mention that, if you don't like some of the ingredients listed here, you can swap them for other Keto pantry items. Regarding your fridge, you should have the following:

- Butter (grass-fed if possible).

- Eggs (free-range and pastured are superior).

- Cheese of your preference. Aged cheddar and mozzarella are good picks, but there are plenty Keto-friendly cheeses.

- Ground beef, whole poultry (the thighs are particularly good for Keto), or both.

- Sour cream, plain yogurt, or Greek yogurt (better than plain yogurt for Keto).

- Heavy cream, or full-fat coconut milk. You can have both as well.

- Cream cheese and mayonnaise.

- Coconut aminos (perfect for salad dressings along with avocado oil).

- Hot sauce (if you're into the flavor).

Maybe you won't use some of these, but this is a great place to start if you need a reference—Some recipes might require a particular ingredient not listed here, but most will include some of these ingredients.

Some common ingredients perish very fast, need to be fresh, or are finicky to store for an extended period, so each meal prep session should take this into consideration.

For example, avocados are a mainstay in several Keto recipes, but they expire quickly after being cut.

This should cover your tools and pantry. For now, focus on getting some proper containers to store your meals and ingredients. This is very important!

You shouldn't just stuff Tupperware bowls with food—doing so will result in copious amounts of stale food. More about containers in the next page.

Storage

The best kind of containers are the ones with divisions for each part of the meal, otherwise you risk cross contamination from one food to the other.

Look for air-tight containers, with air-tight divided section. The result is fresher, crispier, and of course, tastier meals.

You *probably* don't have many containers that accommodate to these characteristics. So, if you've got buy any, make sure that they're also:

- Same-sized: Ease of storing, and better for stacking, saving room in your fridge.

- Transparent: Clear containers will allow you to see what's inside without having to open then; very convenient, and if you're dealing with multiple meals it will become invaluable!

- General safety: Your containers should be freezer, dishwasher, and microwavable safe. Remember to *carefully* check for these details, failure to do so will lead to disappointment once they start breaking apart.

These are pretty solid and somewhat standard counselling for anyone buying food containers, but should consider getting BPA-Free containers as well. The details are somewhat technical, but it never hurts to share some information.

BPA stands for Bisphenol-A, a chemical with estrogenic activity (imitates estrogen); it can potentially affect the health of mammals, including us.

The chemical has been used for decades, but it has been declining in use due to the concerns regarding its safety. It's not the root of all evil, but avoiding it won't do any harm, not if you pick something more harmful at least.

Alternatively, you could opt for glass food containers. They come in different shapes, are safe for almost all operations, and don't include plastic chemicals. They're nonetheless more expensive and often bulkier—It's a matter of compromises, but it comes down to preferences.

Preparing Meals - The Proper Way

We're not going to discuss the Keto recipes yet. First, let's go over *how* you're going to approach meal prep.

Plan Menus

You can save time by having your menus defined *before* heading to the oven. In this book, I will provide you with four menus, for four weeks. But! You can mix 'n' match dishes however you like it! (As long as your picks comply with the Keto diet, of course)

You should try to give your menus some consistency, however.

What I mean by this is that each month should follow the schedule of the previous, and each week should have certain meals in specific days—Maybe it's just me, but if you really like eating fattier cuts of meat, you could have them every Friday or Wednesday, it will greatly enhance your motivation!

Based on your menus, you can make your shopping lists faster than before, and in turn, this will allow you to capitalize on sales and coupons!

Optimize

Seriously, you can cook *a lot* of things at the same time! You need to learn how to use all the tools at your disposal at the maximum of their abilities.

For instance, your oven space should be used to its fullest capacity—Don't go placing one thing after the other, you can put many! Make use of multiple oven trays, and don't forget you can use aluminum foil to make dividers within an oven tray.

During your prep session, go for the foods that take the longest to cook first, such as proteins, whole grains, and beans. That way you can do your multitasking from the start: chop vegetables and fruits as your foods bake, or wash your greens and eggs as your food bubbles on the stovetop.

If you'd rather *not* pre-crook proteins, you can marinate poultry and fish. You'll just have to pop them into the oven before eating.

Try preparing your recipes in a way that you *always* have extra portions—you never know when they're going to save the day, or the next week.

Storing

Proper storing is the difference between having your meals crispy and fresh, or having them go stale before you get to eat.

Perhaps one of the most common causes for food going stale is forgetting about it—really, the fastest way to lose a stew is storing it on the back of your fridge inside an opaque container.

There are many ways you can avoid this problem. First, you could label all your prepped items with a date or a name. You should rotate your containers as you get your food in order to keep things up front. The perishables should always be stored at the very front, that way you won't be forgetting them.

Don't forget that different foods react differently to freezing and refrigeration. Frozen food might lose its texture after a long time, but you can still use it in some recipes, like soups and stews.

Refer to the following lists if you're not sure about how long you can store your foods. When refrigerating at 40°F (4°C) or lower:

- Cooked *ground* poultry or beef: 1 to 2 days.

- Cooked *whole* poultry, meats, fish; soups and stews: 3 to 4 days.

- Cooked beans: 5 days.

- Hardboiled eggs; chopped vegetables (if stored in an airtight container): 1 week.

- Opened *soft* cheese: 2 weeks.

- Opened *hard* cheese: 5 to 6 weeks.

- When freezing at -0°F (-18°C):

- Soups and stews; cooked beans: 2 to 3 months.

- Cooked or ground poultry and meat: 3 to 6 months.

- Berries and chopped fruits (stored in a freezer bag): 6 to 8 months.

- Vegetables (if previously blanched, 3 to 5 minutes): 8 to 12 months.

To Resume

Meal prep refers to the preparation of meals ahead of time; the food of the week is prepared in one or two designated days, and this allows you to save time, but it also gives you more control over *what* you're eating—for that reason alone, most dieters go with meal prepping, as it allows them to minimize their weekly workload, and it helps prevent cravings, emergencies, or mistakes: factors that constantly throw diets into disarray.

Besides this, meal prepping cuts food costs as it will stop you from eating outside, which isn't only expensive but unhealthy.

Generally, meal prep demands only the foods you're going to prepare, a collection of appropriate containers, a couple of free hours, and dedication.

It is *very* simple to do, as it is just cooking and preparing foods, albeit in a more controlled and systematic manner.

By making menus and corresponding shopping lists, you can engage almost any diet with the utmost efficiency.

In turn, you will recover the precious time you spend preparing foods day after day to do other things you want to do, or spend time with your loved ones!

To meal prep, you just need to pick a day and settle to prepare foods for a few hours—proper techniques, multitasking, and organized storage will ensure you spend less time cooking and more time living, without having to worry about the kitchen anymore.

You will receive several meal menus for your Keto diet in the next chapter. You're absolutely free—and even encouraged—to make your own combinations and measurements.

However, the book assumes that you will follow a modified Keto diet, which is not as strict as the traditional, in order to make a smooth transition.

Tips and explanations behind the choices are provided for you to make your own adjustments, should you desire.

Chapter 3

Keto Meal Prep

So! You've made it this far. You know how the Keto diet works, you know how and why you should be a meal prepper, but you still don't know some delicious Keto recipes. It is time we fix that problem!

Writing down what are your specific macronutrient goals (namely proteins, fats, and carbs) will help you remember what you're aiming for, and you should *always* factor that when choosing the recipes.

For the purposes of the following guides, however, we will cover a less-restricting Keto diet.

You shouldn't worry *too much* about the macronutrients, not until you've tried the following meals at least.

Week #1 – Chicken, Cheese, And Bacon

Let's start with a few easy recipes to cover a week—nothing fancy here, just something tasty for you to keep your body running as you strive for Ketosis.

You will chop, cook, and freeze a lot of chicken and bacon.

Preparing your foods during the week will be super simple: just get your things out of the fridge/freezer, reheat, add a few extra touches, and enjoy.

This week's recipes will include:

- Breakfast: Chicken & Egg Sandwich (recipe #4)

- Lunch: Cheese Chicken Burger (recipe #5)

- Dinner: Chicken and Bacon Stuffed Avocado (recipe #6)

- Snacks: Egg & Cheese Chips (recipe #7)

For this week's meal prep, you will need the following ingredients:

- Dried spices: oregano, basil, bay leaves (optional), thyme, parsley, marjoram, savory (alternatively, sage).

- Condiments: salt, pepper, garlic salt (alternatively, garlic powder), onion powder.

- Dressings, fats, and oils: mayonnaise, mustard, avocado oil.

- Proteins: chicken and bacon.

- Dairy: cheddar cheese.

- Vegetables and fruits: avocado, Dill pickles, onions, tomatoes.

Note: The mentioned ingredients aren't "set in stone." Feel free to change them up for whatever you want as long as they're Keto-friendly and interchangeable with the ingredient you want replace.

During your chosen meal prep day, you will do the following:

- For future preparations: Prepare a Keto Seasoning Blend. You can find how in recipe #1. Make sure you store it in an air-tight container in your spice cabinet or other place at room-temperature.

- For breakfast: Prepare, cook, and store 14 Chicken & Bacon Patties in an air-tight container in the freezer. You can find how in recipe #2.

- For lunch: Prepare, cook, and store 7 grilled chicken breasts in an air-tight container in the freezer. You can find how in recipe #3.

- For dinner: Prepare, cook, and store 7 cups of cubed grilled chicken breasts in an air-tight container in the freezer. You can find how in recipe #3.

- Chop and store 21 slices of cheddar cheese. Make sure you store them in an air-tight container in the fridge.

- For snacks: You can use bits of cheese instead of shredded cheese.

Week #2 – Chicken, Bacon, And Veggies

It has been a long week. You've been eating chicken and bacon patties, stuffed avocados, and chicken and cheese burgers.

I believe that a few dishes of healthy salads—drizzled with delicious homemade dressings—accompanied by servings of chicken and bacon are a much-needed change of pace.

This week's recipes will include:

- Breakfast: Bacon & Scrambled Eggs (recipe #9)

- Lunch: Caprese Chicken Bites (recipe #10) *or* Grilled Chicken & Bacon Salad (recipe #11) *or* Keto Roast Chicken (recipe #8)

- Dinner: Caprese Chicken Bites (recipe #10) *or* Grilled Chicken & Bacon Salad (recipe #11) *or* Keto Roast Chicken (recipe #8)

- Snack: Keto Trail-Mix (recipe #11)

For this week's meal prep, you will need the following ingredients:

- Dried spices: basil leaves. You will need the Keto seasoning blend you made in the first week as well.

- Condiments: salt, pepper.

- Dressings, fats, and oils: mustard, white wine vinegar, olive or avocado oil.

- Proteins: chicken thighs, whole chicken, pork, and bacon.

- Dairy: mozzarella cheese.

- Vegetables and fruits: avocado, onions, tomatoes.

- Any sugar substitute. Swerve or Stevia works well.

Note: The mentioned ingredients aren't "set in stone." Feel free to change them up for whatever you want as long as they're Keto-friendly and interchangeable with the ingredient you want replace.

During your chosen meal prep day, you will do the following:

- For lunch: Prepare and bake a whole chicken. Chop into 8 pieces and store in an air-tight container in the freezer. You can find how at recipe #8.

- For lunch and/or dinner: Prepare, cook, and store 3 grilled chicken breasts in an air-tight container in the freezer. You can find how in recipe #3.

- For lunch and/or dinner: Prepare, cook, and store 3 cups of cubed grilled chicken breasts in an air-tight container in the freezer. You can find how in recipe #3.

- For lunch and/or dinner: Prepare, cook, and store 195g of pork slices in an air-tight container in the freezer—just coat with a teaspoon of olive/avocado oil, apply salt to both sides, and cook in oven set to broil. Cook until golden brown and crispy, 20 to 30 minutes.

- For lunch and/or dinner: Chop leafy greens for salad (such as lettuce or spinach). Submerge in water (clean and cold) for 5 to 10 minutes.

    Drain the water, and let the greens dry completely. Store the leafy greens in an air-tight container, or Ziploc bag, in the refrigerator—It is absolutely important you remove any bad pieces from the container, they *will* spoil the rest.

Week #3 – Chicken, Eggs, And Veggies

Let's double down on the chicken and veggies!

Chicken and bacon is good enough, but what about chicken salads with tasty salads and delicious dressings? Let's spice things up with several chicken recipes and a flavorful breakfast.

This week's recipes will include:

- Breakfast: Cauliflower & Sunny Side Up Egg Hash (recipe #16) *or* Cajun Cauliflower Egg Hash (recipe #17)

- Lunch: Lemon & Thyme Chicken Cubes (recipe #13) *or* Cajun Rub Chicken Cubes (recipe #14) *or* Southwestern Chicken Cubes (recipe #15)

- Dinner: Lemon & Thyme Chicken Cubes (recipe #13) *or* Cajun Rub Chicken Cubes (recipe #14) *or* Southwestern Chicken Cubes (recipe #15)

- Snack: Keto Pinwheels (recipe #19)

For this week's meal prep, you will need the following ingredients:

- Dried spices: thyme, basil, cilantro, oregano.

- Condiments: salt, pepper, red pepper flakes, paprika, chili powder, onion powder, Cajun, cayenne, cumin.

- Dressings, fats, and oils: mustard, white wine vinegar, olive or avocado oil, MCT oil, Dijon mustard, mayonnaise.

- Proteins: chicken thighs, pepperoni, pastrami.

- Dairy: cream cheese.

- Vegetables and fruits: avocado, onions, tomatoes, cauliflower.

Note: The mentioned ingredients aren't "set in stone." Feel free to change them up for whatever you want as long as they're Keto-friendly and interchangeable with the ingredient you want replace.

During your chosen meal prep day, you will do the following:

- For breakfast: Prepare, cook, and store 4 servings of Cauliflower & Sunny Side Up Egg Hash in an air-tight container in the refrigerator (not the freezer). Find how in recipe #16.

- For breakfast: Prepare, cook, and store 3 servings of Cajun Cauliflower Egg Hash in an air-tight container in the refrigerator (not the freezer). Find how in recipe #17.

- Prepare, cook, and store several cups of the three chicken cube recipes provided: Lemon & Thyme Chicken Cubes (recipe #13), Cajun Rub Chicken Cubes (recipe #14), *and* Southwestern Chicken Cubes (recipe #15). Remember to store in an air-tight container in the freezer. Check the respective recipes to prepare them.

- For lunch and/or dinner: Chop leafy greens for salad (such as lettuce or spinach). Submerge in water (clean and cold) for 5 to 10 minutes. Drain the water, and let the greens dry completely.

  Store the leafy greens in an air-tight container, or Ziploc bag, in the refrigerator—It is absolutely important you remove any bad pieces from the container, they *will* spoil the rest.

- There are several garnishes you can prepare for the salads: You can chop and store several cheese cubes; you can prepare, cook, and store several slices of pork to slice into cubes; and lastly, you can prepare and store a Keto-friendly salad dressing, you can find how in recipe #19.

Week #4 – Shrimps, Turkey, and Eggs

Let's top it off with some ingredients you haven't used yet: Shrimps and turkey.

Seafood is a delicacy for many, but beyond that, it is impressively good for your health and specially Keto.

This week's recipes will include:

- Breakfast: Keto Meat Eggs & Veggies (recipe #22)

- Lunch: Keto Shrimps (recipe #20) or Keto Thai Turkey (recipe #21)

- Dinner: Keto Shrimps (recipe #20) or Keto Thai Turkey (recipe #21)

- Snack: Keto Caramelized Chips (recipe #23)

For this week's meal prep, you will need the following ingredients:

- Spices: cinnamon.

- Condiments: salt, pepper, ground cumin, onion and garlic powder, Thai red curry paste.

- Dressings, fats, and oils: Olive (or avocado oil), rice vinegar, soy sauce, lime juice, sesame oil.

- Proteins: shrimps, ground turkey, bacon (or sausages, or salami).

- Dairy: cheddar cheese.

- Vegetables and fruits: garlic, onion, green onions, green peppers.

Note: The mentioned ingredients aren't "set in stone." Feel free to change them up for whatever you want as long as they're Keto-friendly and interchangeable with the ingredient you want replace.

During your chosen meal prep day, you will do the following:

- For lunch/dinner: Prepare, cook, and store 40 shrimps in an air-tight container in the freezer. You can find how in recipe #20.

- For lunch/dinner: Prepare and cook 7 Keto Thai Turkey Wrap fillings with their sauce. Store 3 to 4 in the refrigerator, and store the remaining in the freezer. You can find how at recipe #21.

- For breakfast: Prepare, cook, and store 7 portions of scrambled eggs. Prepare, cook, and store 7 portions of the cooked vegetables of your preference (broccoli and mushrooms for example). Chop and store 7 portions of meat (could be bacon, salami, sausages) in the freezer.

- Dice cheddar cheese into cubes and store for the salads you will be eating alongside your meals. A few cups. You can prepare a dressing for the salads too. Find how in recipe #19.

- For lunch and/or dinner: Chop leafy greens for salad (such as lettuce or spinach). Submerge in water (clean and cold) for 5 to 10 minutes. Drain the water, and let the greens dry completely.

  Store the leafy greens in an air-tight container, or Ziploc bag, in the refrigerator—It is absolutely important you remove any bad pieces from the container, they *will* spoil the rest.

To Resume

All these weeks are merely *examples* of how you could handle your meal prep. They may suit your needs and taste, but, if they don't, that's alright! With the proposed foods, you can prepare a plethora of dishes, not just the recommended ones.

In the following chapter, you will learn different recipes to prepare your breakfast, lunch, dinner, and snacks for the week. However, none of these are "set in stone."

You're free to come up with your own creative combinations! Just use *any* of the Keto-friendly foods available. Whenever you're unsure about particular foods, remember: the higher the carbs, the farther it has to be from your diet.

Many of the recipes can include additional garnishes, and I give you a short list of suggestions. Again, you can add anything you want, as long as it doesn't mess your daily nutritional intake.

One last thing to have in mind: Using a kitchen scale is not necessary, but it allows you to know *precisely* the distribution of nutrients you're consuming—it can be a huge help if you want to further tweak your daily intake.

Recipe #1 – Keto Seasoning Blend

Store-bought seasoning blends are a big help. But, as is this the case with most common purchasable products, they're made with carb-based fillers like corn starch.

If you've got a stocked spice cabinet, getting your meat or sauce seasoned *just* the way you want it while being Keto-friendly is possible, albeit time consuming—you have to juggle different spice jars *every single time* you prepare meat or sauce.

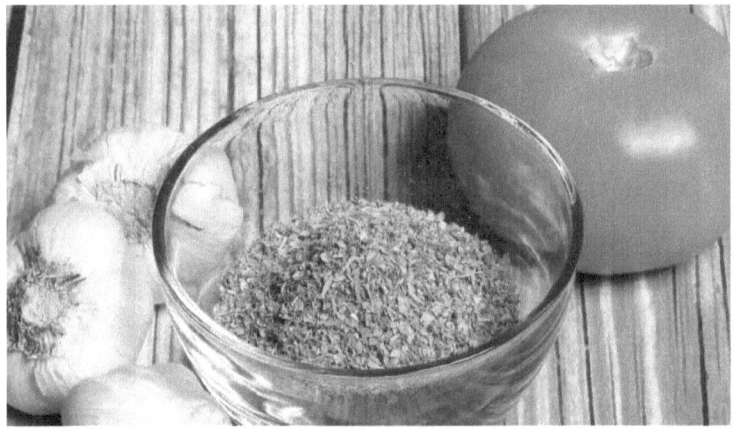

With but a single trip to the spice cabinet, you will prepare a homemade Italian-style seasoning blend for all your Keto recipes.

Doing this in advance will save you *a lot* of time during meal prep. The quantities are suitable for a decent batch, and the blend can work basically in any recipe that calls for an Italian seasoning.

Ingredients

- 2 Tablespoons of dried oregano
- 2 Tablespoons of dried basil
- 1 Tablespoon of dried thyme
- 1 Tablespoon of dried rosemary
- 1 Tablespoon of dried parsley
- 2 Teaspoons of dried savory (alternatively, a teaspoon of dried sage and a teaspoon of dried marjoram)
- 1 Teaspoon of red pepper flakes
- 1/2 Teaspoon of garlic salt (alternatively, garlic powder)
- 1/2 Teaspoon of onion powder
- Optional: 2 Dried bay leaves (about 1/2 crushed)
- Optional: 1 Tablespoon of dried marjoram

Preparation

1. Combine all the ingredients in a small bowl, and mix thoroughly until well combined.

   Remember you can swap some of the ingredients or their quantities according to your preference—Be aware, it will change the flavor and whether or not you can use it in certain recipes that require Italian seasoning.

2. If you've got a food processor: Pulse about 5 to 10 times to get a finer consistency, unless you prefer the irregular texture.

3. Store in an air-tight container, room temperature. Probably best to put it in your spice cabinet with a label.

Recipe #2 – Chicken & Bacon Patties

Delicious, quick to make, and easy to store. Is there anything else we can ask from these patties? You can bake them, but you could also pan-fry them in an oil of your choosing (coconut oil is great) to add a crispier texture, as well as hints of other flavors.

They're perfectly safe in the fridge—just reheat them each time you need a quick meal and you're done!

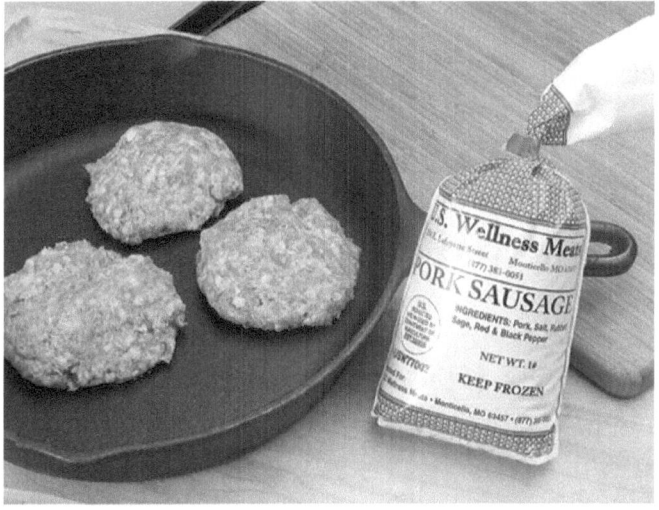

Feel free to omit the eggs if you'd prefer to, but I recommend you add them to the mix: it makes the patties tastier and moister.

Ingredients

- 1 1/4 lbs. of ground chicken (alternatively, 2 large chicken breasts. The ground chicken is better for Keto)

- 2 to 3 Slices of bacon, broken and cooked into small bits (feel free to adjust the bacon ratio)
- 1 Whisked egg
- 2 Tablespoons of Keto seasoning blend (recipe #1)
- 2 Teaspoons of garlic powder
- 2 Teaspoons of onion powder
- Salt and pepper to taste

Preparation

1. Start by preheating the oven to 425°F (220°C). Mix all the ingredients together until well combined. Alternatively, food process all the ingredients together.

2. Make 14 thin patties—about 1/2-inch thick—from the meat mixture. Line a baking tray with foil (you won't have to wash the baking tray after).

3. Bake the patties for about 20 minutes; the internal temperature of the patty nearer to the middle of the tray should be around 170°F (76°C) when checked with a meat thermometer.

   Alternatively, you can pan-fry them in an oil of your choosing to add hints of other flavors, besides a crispier textures, although that will take more than 20 minutes.

4. Let them cool, and store inside an air-tight container in the fridge or freezer—preferably the latter if you intend to make lots of the for the week during Sunday. Reheat in skillet or microwave before eating.

Recipe #3 – Grilled Chicken Breast

A recipe for grilling chicken breasts? What, do you think I just got out of my mother's house?

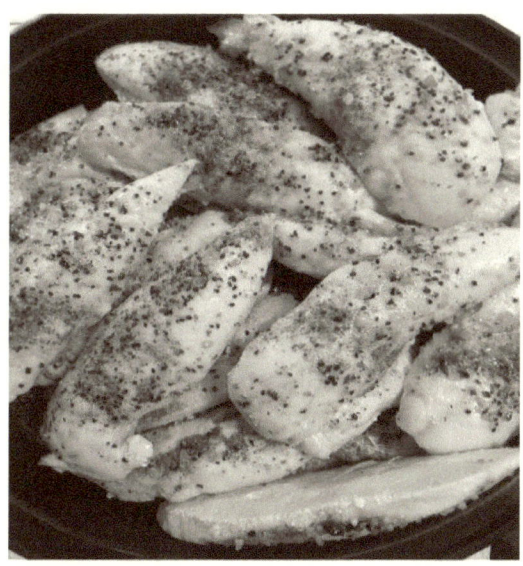

Far from it! I know grilling chicken is *usually* the first thing one learns when cooking. However, there's a better, Keto-friendlier, way of grilling chicken breasts, and it will help you in the following recipes!

Ingredients

- The amount of chicken breasts you want to cook (Make sure they're boneless and skinless)
- 2 Teaspoons of olive oil (alternatively, avocado oil)
- 1 Tablespoon of Keto seasoning blend (recipe #1)
- Salt and pepper to taste

Preparation

1. Get your chicken breasts out of the freezer, and let them thaw.

2. Once thawed, season well on both sides with salt and pepper. Then, season the chicken breasts with the Keto seasoning blend. Turn on the grill, let it heat, and then add the oil.

3. Add the chicken breasts and cook until the sides turn white. Flip them to other side, and cook until the internal temperature of the chicken breasts read about 160°-165°F. You can store them, or you can dice them into cubes.

Recipe #4 – Chicken & Egg Sandwich

I've never been a fan of fast food myself, but I do know a lot of people who go crazy over McMuffins—I can understand their appeal, however: round patties, round bread, melty cheese. Simplicity is the highest form of sophistication.

Nonetheless, I think we're all aware by know (I hope we are) that fast food is downright *unhealthy*, there's no debate about it. You will want to stay pretty far from any kind of fast food during the Keto diet; that's not to say you cannot enjoy your own Keto twist of the McMuffin though!

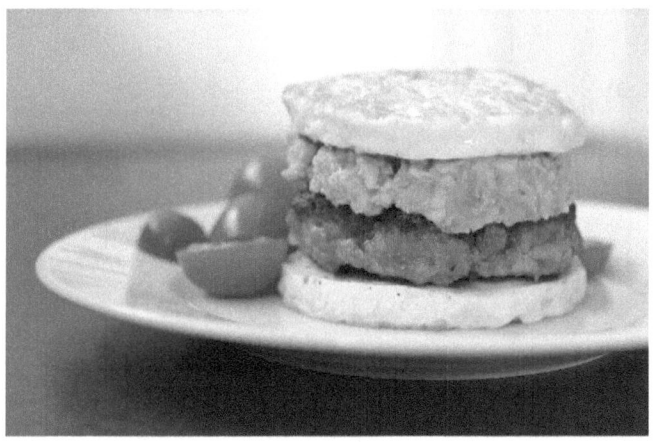

Plain bacon & eggs is tasty enough, that much is true. But this recipe adds bells and whistles to an otherwise godly combination for breakfast.

Note: If you want to make perfectly round shaped eggs, you will need a few mason jar rings (or silicone egg molds). You can skip this part if you don't mind.

Ingredients

- 1 Tablespoon of butter
- 2 Large eggs (free-range and pastured if you can)
- 1 Tablespoon of mayonnaise
- 2 Chicken & Bacon patties (recipe #2)
- 2 Slices of cheddar cheese (sharp if possible)
- 2 – 3 Slices of avocado

Preparation

1. Heat butter in a large skillet, medium heat. Lightly oil your mason jar rings (or egg molds), and place them into the pan. You can skip this part if you don't have any rings or molds.

2. Crack the eggs into the rings, break the yolks with a fork, and whisk gently. Cover and cook for 3 to 4 minutes. Reheat your patties in a skillet or microwave as your eggs are cooked. Remove the eggs from the rings with a spatula and a tong.

   If going without the rings: crack the eggs into the pan, break the yolks, and whisk gently. Scoop out as normal.

3. Place an egg on a plate, top it with half the tablespoon of mayonnaise, and place one of the patties. Top the patty with a slice of cheese, and one to two slices of avocado.

4. Place the second patty on top of the avocado and cheese, and top it with the remaining cheese and avocado.

5. Spread the remaining mayonnaise on the second egg, and put it on top the cheese to finish the sandwich. You're ready to enjoy your breakfast!

A little tip to keep avocados fresh for longer:

- Cut an avocado in half, and cut two handfuls of large onion chunks. Place a handful of onion chunks in an airtight container, and an avocado half, face up, on top, and seal it.

  Repeat the process with the other avocado half—This will keep the avocado fresh and ready to be sliced for the entire week.

Note: You can always choose to have a different breakfast—This is just a suggestion you can follow. If you'd rather have a different dish, go for it! It simply has to be both Keto-friendly and satiating.

Recipe #5 – Chicken Cheese Burger

Technically, you cannot eat bread in the Keto diet—that doesn't mean you've got to enjoy your burgers without buns.

You've got two options for buns here: Portobello mushroom caps or lettuce—I prefer the mushroom caps myself, they're tastier and crispier!

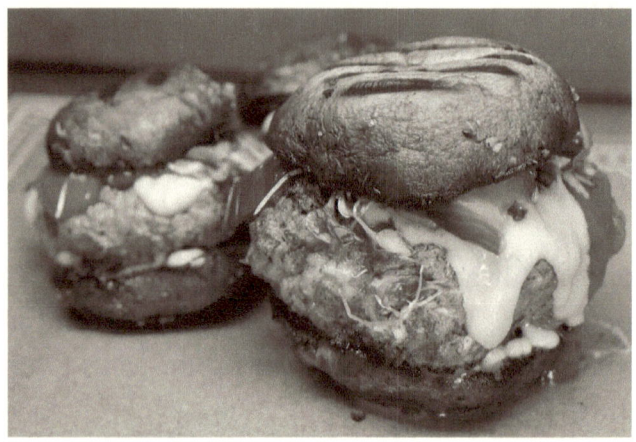

A single Portobello mushroom packs more potassium than a banana; perfect if you're dealing with any of the side-effects of ketosis.

Ingredients

- 1 Teaspoon of salt
- 1 Teaspoon of pepper (black pepper is great)
- 1 Tablespoon of avocado oil
- 1 Slices of cheddar cheese (sharp if possible)
- 1 Chicken Milanese

For buns

- 1 to 2 Portobello mushroom caps, per burger (destemmed, rinsed, and dabbed dry)
- Lettuce, as many as you need to make a solid bun
- Something of your preference that can be used for buns

Pick any and as many garnishes as you want

- Sliced dill pickles (I love them!)
- Alfalfa sprouts
- A couple of avocado slices
- Lettuce
- Sliced onions or tomatoes (not too many)

Preparation

1. Get your patties out of the freezer, and let them thaw for a moment while you prepare the rest of the ingredients for the burgers. You can thaw the patties in the microwave, or by putting the frozen meat in a plastic bag and submerging it in cold water. The former is faster.

2. Heat the avocado oil in a large pan, medium heat. Add the mushroom caps and cook about 3 to 4 minutes, each side. Remove the mushroom caps from the heat and add your patties. Cook for 4 minutes each side. Add the cheese on top each patty, cover with a lid, and let the cheese melt for a minute.

3. Place one of the mushroom caps in a plate, then a patty. Add some of your garnishes, then the other patty. Add

some of your remaining garnishes, and then top it with the remaining mushroom cap.

The recipe is very modular; you can use a single mushroom cap instead of two, or forego them altogether for a lettuce bed; you can also opt for one or three patties instead of two if you'd prefer. I recommend you layer the ingredients like I did to enhance flavor and texture.

Depending on the garnishes—you can opt for garnishes not mentioned in the list, as long as they're Keto-friendly—you can clean, chop, and/or store them in their corresponding places (spice cabinet, fridge, freezer, etc.).

Note: You can always choose to have a different lunch—This is just a suggestion you can follow. If you'd rather have a different dish, go for it! It simply has to be both Keto-friendly and satiating.

Recipe #6 – Chicken & Bacon Stuffed Avocado

Dinner is very important to me. Nothing makes me feel better at the end of a long day of work than a nice meal—By nice I don't simply refer to a tasty meal, it also has to be light on the stomach!

Since we're going all out on the chicken and bacon, let's top our day with a delicious avocado, stuffed with a bounty of chicken, bacon, and slices of onion and tomato.

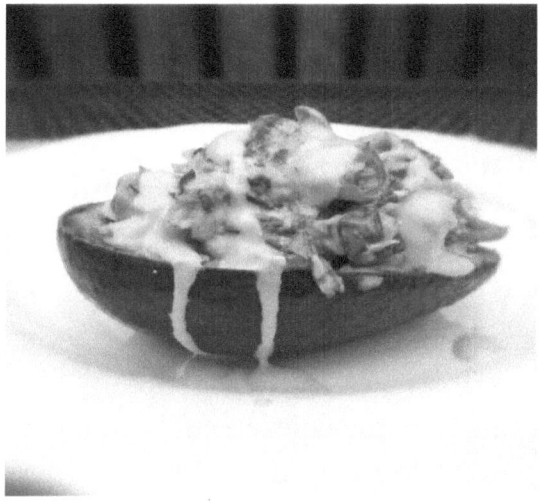

While some Keto dieters stay away from tomatoes and onions, you can add a few slices of each as long as you keep it low.

If you'd like to better gauge how much tomatoes and onions you can eat, 100g of tomatoes have 3.89g of carbs (2.69g net), and 100g of onions have 9.34g of carbs (7.64g net).

Ingredients

- 1 Cup of chicken cubes
- 3 Slices of bacon
- 1 Avocados
- Seasoning to taste.
- 1 Tablespoon of mayonnaise

Pick any and as many garnishes as you want

- 1 Cup of sliced onions
- 1 Cup of sliced tomatoes
- 1 Cup of sliced Dill pickles
- Tiny slices of cheddar cheese

Preparation

1. Get your chicken cubes out of the freezer and let them thaw while you prepare the rest of the ingredients for the stuffed avocados.

   You can thaw the chicken cubes in the microwave, or by putting the frozen poultry in a plastic bag and submerging it in cold water. The former is faster.

2. Grill the bacon strips, about 2 to 3 minutes per side. They should be pretty crispy. Set them aside, and dice them into small bits. Reheat the chicken cubes.

3. Mix cubed chicken, bacon, tomatoes, onions, and any additional garnish and seasoning you want in a

medium bowl (I like adding sliced pickles, and a pinch of salt and pepper).

4. Add the tablespoon of mayonnaise, mixing it evenly into the rest of the ingredients. Slice the avocados in half, discarding the pit, and then pile the bowl's content on top of each avocado half.

Note: You can always choose to have a different dinner—This is just a suggestion you can follow. If you'd rather have a different dish, go for it! It simply has to be both Keto-friendly and satiating.

Recipe #7 – Egg & Cheese Chips

If you liked potato chips you're going to love these low-carbs crispy cheese chips. They're extremely easy to make, satisfying, and you can keep them in your pack for the entire day!

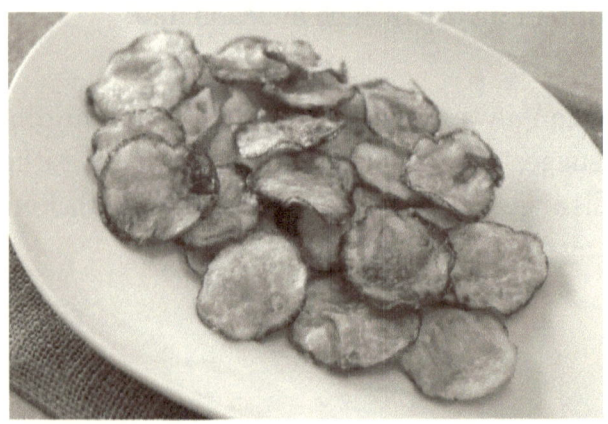

Believe me when I tell you that you won't be missing potato chips after trying them!

Ingredients

- 4 egg whites
- Half cup of shredded cheddar cheese
- 1 Teaspoon of salt
- 1 Teaspoon of pepper
- Optional: 1 Teaspoon of garlic
- Optional: 1 Teaspoon of dried rosemary

You will need either avocado or olive oil to grease the muffin tray. I suggest avocado oil, but you can go for olive oil.

Preparation

1. Start by preheating your oven to 400°F (204°C). Grease your muffin tray with either olive or avocado oil. Add the 4 egg whites and seasoning of choice into a bowl, whisk well. A pinch of garlic, salt, pepper, and rosemary do the trick, but you can get creative!

2. Spoon half tablespoons of your egg mixture into each muffin compartment—ideally until you have a thin layer covering the bottom. The thinner the layer, the crispier the chip.

3. Top each compartment with shredded cheese (or just tiny bits of cheese), just a bit, not a handful. Make sure the cheese isn't touching the edges of the compartment, it tends to stick to the sides. You can use a knife or a spatula to do so.

4. Baking time will largely depend on how thick your egg mixture is—it should take between 10 to 20 minutes; alternatively, bake until the edges have browned.

5. Remove the chips from the pan and you're ready to enjoy! Enjoy them as a side-dish, or prepare them in the morning and bring them to work as snacks.

Note: You can always choose to have a different snack—This is just a suggestion you can follow. If you'd rather have a different dish, go for it! It simply has to be both Keto-friendly and satiating.

Recipe #8 – Keto Roast Chicken

This delicious baked chicken makes a total of 8 servings, and comes out with next to no carbs.

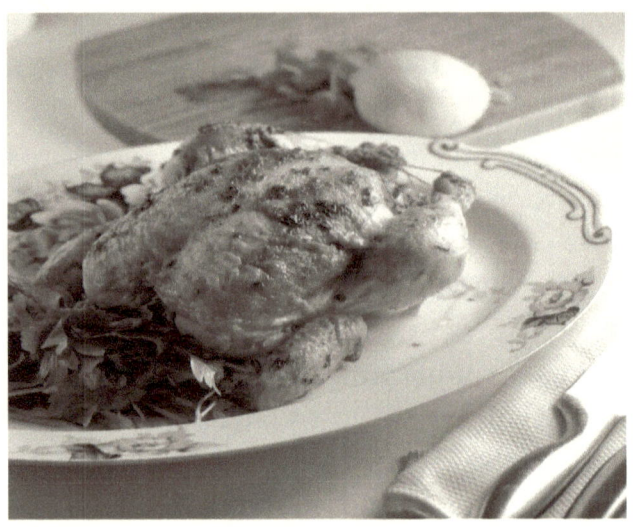

It takes some time to prepare and cook, but it's worth every minute given how many portions you can get.

Ingredients

- 1 Whole chicken
- 1/3 Cup of soy sauce
- 1 Tablespoon of Swerve (or any other sugar substitute)
- 6 Slices of ginger
- 1 Teaspoon of Keto Seasoning Blend
- Any Keto-friendly vegetables you wish to stuff the chicken with.

Preparation

1. Add soy sauce, Swerve (or any other sugar substitute), and ginger slices in a large Ziploc bag. Make sure it's well combined. Remove the giblets inside the chicken, and spoon half the teaspoon of Keto seasoning blend inside.

2. Place the chicken inside the bag, and turn it to full coat. Be sure to marinade overnight, and try to turn it occasionally.

3. Preheat oven to 350°F (175°C), and place chicken over a baking sheet. Make sure you tuck the wings under the chicken, and then cut some holes near the bottom of the chicken to secure its legs.

4. Roast the chicken with whatever vegetables you wish to serve for 20 minutes. Then, baste the chicken with the grease that has collected below it. Cook for 20 minutes.

   Baste again. Repeat until the chicken has cooked for an hour—As you do this process, place the rest of the marinade in a small pot on the stove. Cook it down so that it thickens up, and whisk often.

5. Once the chicken is done cooking, start basting it with the thickened marinade every 10 minutes for half an hour. Ideally use a thermometer to check that the chicken reached 165°F (74°C).

The chicken is done, you're free to cut it into 8 servings—A serving of this delicious chicken is great alongside a green salad with some oil!

Recipe #9 – Bacon & Scrambled Eggs

An old time classic for breakfast. They're as simple and easy to prepare as they get, they're tasty, and they're Keto-friendly.

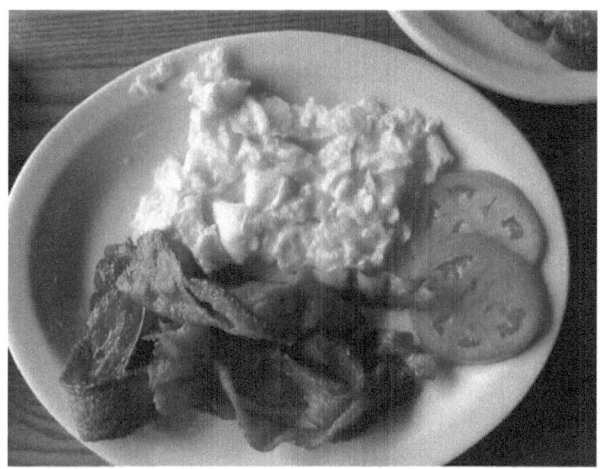

The hardest part about cooking eggs is not letting them overcook, but I got you covered.

One last thing, you're cooking bacon in the oven, not a pan!

Ingredients

- 3 Large eggs (free-range and pastured)
- 1 Tablespoon of butter
- 4 Slices of bacon
- 1 Teaspoon of salt
- 1 Teaspoon of pepper

Note: You can add other ingredients to the dish. Vegetables, slices of cheese, or even more bacon! Just keep the rations moderate, you're striving for a balance of fats, carbs, and proteins, not just proteins!

Preparation

1. Start by preheating your oven to 350°F (175°C). Line bacon slices on a cookie sheet. Pop into oven when its heated. Cook in oven until crispy, about 10 to 15 minutes.

2. Heat your pan, medium-low. Add in butter, and let it melt. Crack and mix the eggs in a bowl, then add them to pan.

3. Don't stir yet. Let them set on the bottom. Stir gently, about 3 to 4 times, to bring the eggs from the bottom to the top.

4. Once they've set to the bottom again, fold the eggs over to ensure the mixture cooks. Add salt and pepper to taste. Remove from pan, and enjoy your breakfast!

Don't forget you can add other garnishes and foods—I like adding *just a few* slices of tomatoes and onions, and two big slices of avocado.

Note: You can always choose to have a different breakfast— This is just a suggestion you can follow. If you'd rather have a different dish, go for it! It simply has to be both Keto-friendly and satiating.

Recipe #10 – Caprese Chicken Bites

Tasty and juicy pan-seared chicken thighs, drizzled with fresh pesto sauce, and topped with tomato and mozzarella cheese— Remind me again what's the boring part of being on a diet!

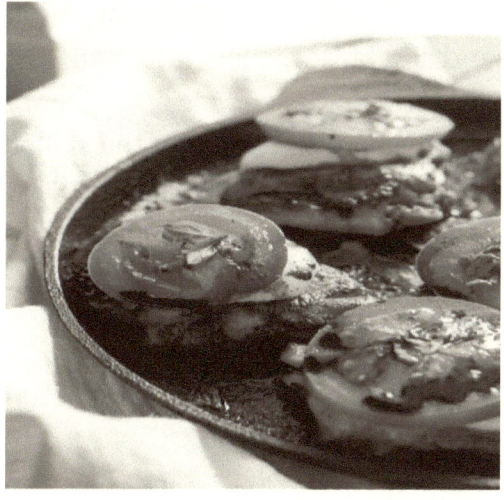

Chicken breasts often come up dry, but the thighs are usually tender and juicy.

Ingredients

- 1/8 Tablespoon of butter
- 1 Grilled chicken thigh
- 1/2 Cup of basil leaves
- 1/8 Cup of olive oil
- 1/8 Cup of pine nuts
- 1 Ounces of sliced tomatoes
- 1 Ounces of sliced mozzarella cheese

Preparation

1. Start by preheating your oven to 350°F (175°C)—Get your chicken breasts out of the freezer, and let them thaw.

2. Preheat a cast iron skillet (any one as long as its oven-safe) and add butter, allow it to melt.

3. Lay the chicken thigh down in the skillet. Let it reheat for a few minutes. Blend basil leaves, olive oil, and pine nuts in a food processor. Season to taste with salt.

4. Turn off the skillet's heat, and spoon the pesto sauce over the chicken thigh. Layer a mozzarella slice, then a tomato.

5. Bake for about 30 minutes—The chicken should be cooked all the way through, and the cheese should be melted and browned.

It is best if you accompany this dish with a serving of salad— use the leafy greens you chopped and stored, as well as a few slices of avocados, onions, and tomatoes, or any other vegetables you'd prefer.

Note: You can always choose to have a different lunch or dinner—This is just a suggestion you can follow. If you'd rather have a different dish, go for it! It simply has to be both Keto-friendly and satiating.

Recipe #11 – Grilled Chicken & Bacon Salad

I love varied flavors and textures in my food—it breaks the monotony of each bite, and makes you feel like you're eating a lot more than what it seems.

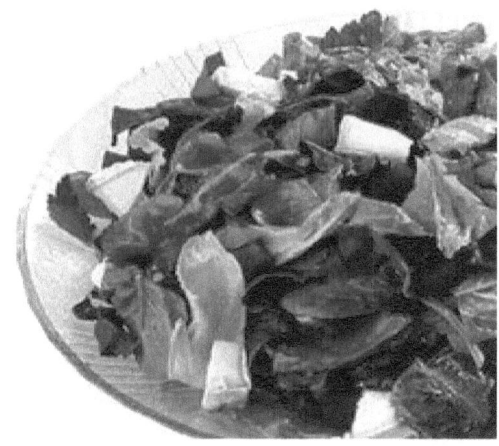

This delicious salad is filled with flavor, aroma, and taste. You can decide what goes in, from the nuts, to the oils. Truly spectacular!

Ingredients

- 65g Pork slices
- 1 Cup of cubed chicken
- 10g Pine nuts
- 1/2 Tablespoon of Swerve (Stevia, or another sugar substitute)
- 20g Mozzarella Cheese (or another cheese of your preference)

- 1/8 Medium pear
- 1/4 Teaspoon of Dijon mustard (yellow mustard works as well)
- 1/4 Teaspoons of wholegrain mustard
- 1 Tablespoon of white wine vinegar
- 1 Teaspoon of olive oil (alternatively, avocado oil)
- 30g Mixed greens (your preference, could be lettuce or spinach)
- Optional: Parmesan cheese to sprinkle at the end

Preparation

1. Get your pork slices and chicken cubes out of the freezer, and let them thaw for a moment. Chop pine nuts into smaller pieces.

2. Heat a pan, medium-high. Add water and Swerve (or another sugar substitute). When Swerve dissolves, add your chopped nuts. Cook for about 5 minutes, until the liquid has thickened and caramelized on the nuts. Set them aside onto a tray to cool.

3. Chop your desired cheese and pear into bite size pieces. Reheat pork slices in oven or pan, preferably oven. Slice them into small pieces after they've cooled a bit. Reheat chicken cubes in oven or pan.

4. Prepare a vinaigrette: add mustards, white wine vinegar, and olive (or avocado) oil into a small bowl. Whisk with a fork until thickened and well combined.

5. Add your salad greens, drizzle the vinaigrette, and top with the sliced pork and cubed chicken. Add nuts, cheese, and pear. I like sprinkling Parmesan cheese before eating.

Feel free to change some of the ingredients—you can drop/swap the nuts, cheese, pear, and mustards. This is only one way to do it!

Note: You can always choose to have a different lunch or dinner—This is just a suggestion you can follow. If you'd rather have a different dish, go for it! It simply has to be both Keto-friendly and satiating.

Recipe #12 – Keto Trail-Mix

I absolutely *adore* trail-mixes. They're non-perishable, they're energy-dense, they're delicious, and they're perfect for almost any kind of lifestyle—They're, however, not Keto-friendly.

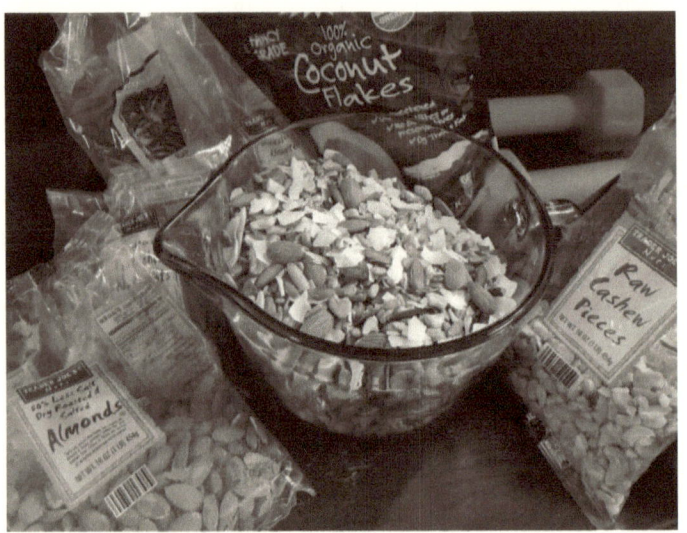

Most of the store-bought packages come with sugar sources such as candies, chocolate chips, or dried fruits. We're going to make our own Keto-friendly mix to power us through the day without all the carbs!

Ingredients

- 1 Cup of roasted peanuts
- 1 Cup of roasted almonds (or pine nuts)
- 1 Cup of pumpkin nuts
- 2 oz. unsweetened coconuts

- 1/2 Cup of currants or raisins (Raisins are a bit high in carb, so use a smaller amount. Currants are better because they pack fewer carbs.

Preparation

1. Mix all of that together in a cup, really!

There's not much to say about this little recipe. Feel free to swap the nuts and seeds for something else entirely, but remember to watch out for the carbs!

Note: You can always choose to have a different snack—This is just a suggestion you can follow. If you'd rather something else, go for it! It simply has to be both Keto-friendly and satiating.

Recipe #13 –Lemon & Thyme Chicken Cubes

This is part of a series of three recipes. *Lemon & Thyme*, *Cajun Rub*, and *Southwestern* Chicken cubes.

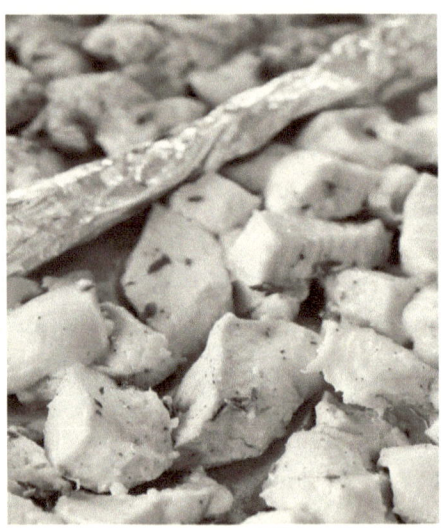

These recipes are fairly simple, so let's cut your meal prep time by doing one simple trick: cover a sheet pan with foil, and then make two sheets of foil into long sticks—use these to separate the sheet pan into thirds, and cook each recipe *at the same time* in the same sheet!

Ingredients

- 1 1/2 lb. boneless and skinless chicken breasts (cubed)
- Zest from half a lemon
- 2 Tablespoons of fresh lemon juice
- 1 Teaspoon of fresh, diced thyme

- 1/2 to 1 Tablespoon of olive oil (alternatively, avocado oil)
- 1/4 Teaspoon of salt (kosher salt or rough sea salt are great)
- 1/4 Teaspoon of ground pepper, fresh
- 1 Small garlic clove, minced

Preparation

1. Mix all the ingredients in a bowl, combine well. Pour over chicken cubes, toss until fully coated.

2. Bake on one of the divisions of the baking sheet, for about 20 minutes at 400°F (200°C).

Recipe #14 —Cajun Rub Chicken Cubes

This is part of a series of three recipes. *Lemon & Thyme*, *Cajun Rub*, and *Southwestern* Chicken cubes.

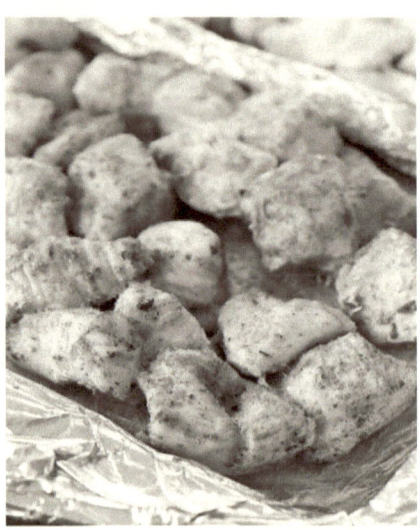

These recipes are fairly simple, so let's cut your meal prep time by doing one simple trick: cover a sheet pan with foil, and then make two sheets of foil into long sticks—use these to separate the sheet pan into thirds, and cook each recipe *at the same time* in the same sheet!

Ingredients

- 1 1/2 lb. boneless and skinless chicken breasts (cubed)
- 1/2 Teaspoon of paprika
- 1/2 Teaspoon of garlic powder
- 1/2 Onion powder
- 1/2 Mexican oregano
- 1/4 Teaspoon of cayenne

- 1/4 Teaspoon of salt (kosher salt or rough sea salt are great)
- 1 Teaspoon of fresh, diced thyme
- 1/2 to 1 Tablespoon of olive oil (alternatively, avocado oil)
- 1/4 Teaspoon of salt (kosher salt or rough sea salt are great)
- 1/8 Teaspoon of red pepper flakes
- 1/4 Teaspoon of ground pepper, fresh
- Olive or avocado oil to drizzle

Preparation

1. Mix all the ingredients, except the oils, in a bowl, combine well. Pour over chicken cubes, toss until fully coated.

2. Sprinkle the mix on the raw chicken cubes. Drizzle with the oil of your preference, and toss. Bake on one of the divisions of the baking sheet, for about 20 minutes at 400°F (200°C).

Recipe #15 –Southwestern Chicken Cubes

This is part of a series of three recipes. *Lemon & Thyme, Cajun Rub*, and *Southwestern* Chicken cubes.

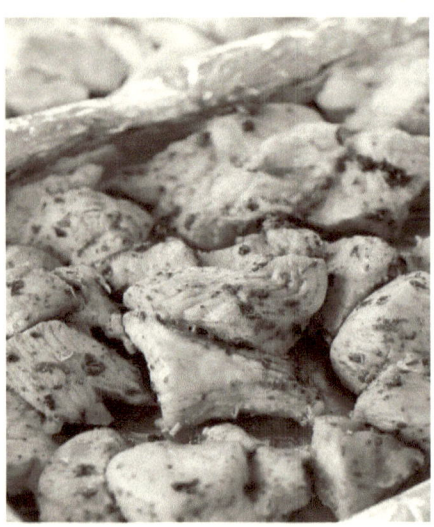

These recipes are fairly simple, so let's cut your meal prep time by doing one simple trick: cover a sheet pan with foil, and then make two sheets of foil into long sticks—use these to separate the sheet pan into thirds, and cook each recipe *at the same time* in the same sheet!

Ingredients

- 1 1/2 lb. boneless and skinless chicken breasts (cubed)
- 1 Small garlic clove, minced
- 1 Tablespoon of fresh lemon juice
- 1/4 Teaspoon of ground cumin

- 1/4 Teaspoon of salt (kosher salt or rough sea salt work great)
- 1/4 Teaspoon of pepper
- 1/4 Teaspoon of Mexican oregano
- 1Tablespoon of fresh cilantro, diced
- 1/2 Tablespoon of olive oil (alternatively, avocado oil)
- 1/4 Teaspoon of chili powder

Preparation

1. Mix all the ingredients in a bowl, combine well. Pour over chicken cubes, toss until fully coated.

2. Bake on one of the divisions of the baking sheet, for about 20 minutes at 400°F (200°C).

Recipe #16 – Cauliflower & Sunny Side Up Egg Hash

Crispy and savory eggs for breakfast are good on their own, but add in a lean hash of pastrami, cauliflower, and peppers and you've got yourself a winning combination for breakfast!

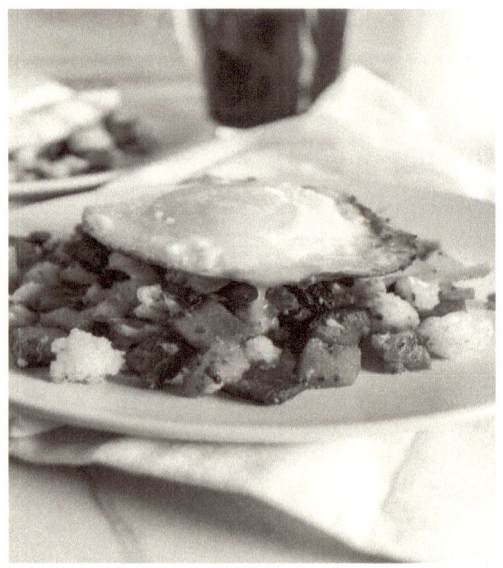

This recipe yields 4 servings of hash you can store for the week. Reheat the hash over a skillet, fry two eggs, and you're ready to breakfast!

Ingredients

- 2 Tablespoons of olive oil (alternatively, avocado oil)
- 2 Tablespoons of salted butter
- 1/2 Large onion, diced about 1/4 inch (1 cup)
- 2 Garlic cloves, diced

- 1/2 Head cauliflower, chopped into 1/4 pieces (4 cups)
- 1/4 Cup of water
- 1/2 lb. of brisket pastrami, diced into 1/4 inch squares
- 1 Cup of green pepper, diced 1/4 inch
- 2 Eggs
- Salt and pepper to taste

Preparation

1. Heat 1 tablespoon of olive (or avocado) oil and 1 tablespoon of butter over a large skillet, medium heat.

2. Add the chopped onion and sauté for 4 minutes. Now, add the diced garlic and sauté for 2 more minutes.

3. Add the finely chopped cauliflower and water to the skillet and sauté. When the water has evaporated—about five minutes in—add the remaining tablespoon of oil and sauté for 10 minutes.

4. Add the diced pastrami and green pepper, sauté for 5 minutes—the pastrami should be heated through, and the peppers should be softened.

5. Taste a bit, and add salt or pepper to taste. If you do, add 1/4 teaspoon at a time. Stir well, and taste again. Turn the heat to low until you plate.

The hash is ready, wait until it cools, and store it in the fridge. When you want to breakfast, you just have to reheat the hash and prepare the eggs like so:

1. Place hash in a skillet, and reheat over medium heat. Sautéing for 5 to 7 minutes.

2. Move to the eggs. Melt the remaining tablespoon of butter in a skillet over medium heat. Add 2 eggs. Fry on one side until the edges are golden and the white is set.

3. It's time to plate. Place a cup of cauliflower hash on a plate, and top with one egg.

Recipe #17 – Cajun Cauliflower Egg Hash

Nothing out of the ordinary here—Just the delicious, lean pastrami, cauliflower and pepper hash you're accustomed to, but with spicy Cajun twist!

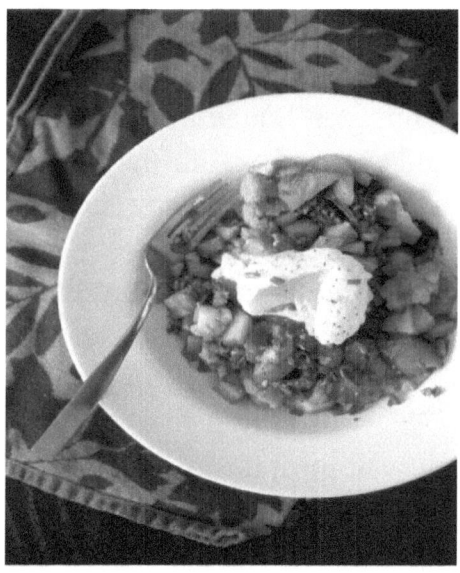

This recipe yields 3 servings of hash you can store for the week. Reheat the hash over a skillet, fry two eggs, and you're ready to breakfast!

Ingredients

- 2 Tablespoon of olive (or avocado) oil (alternatively, ghee)
- 1/2 Onion, chopped into 1/4 inch pieces
- 2 1/2 Tablespoons of garlic, minced
- 1 1/2 lb. of frozen cauliflower, steamed and chopped into small, even chunks)

- 1 Teaspoon of Cajun seasoning
- 12 oz. of shaved red pastrami, chopped into 1" slices
- 1/2 green pepper, chopped into 1/4 inch pieces

Preparation

1. Heat 2 tablespoon of olive (or avocado) oil over a large skillet, medium heat. Add your chopped onions, and sauté for 5 minutes. Squeeze any excess water from your steamed and chopped cauliflower, and add it, sauté for 5 to 10 minutes until it gets crispy and browned.

2. Add Cajun seasoning, and mix well. Add the chopped pastrami and green peppers. Toss and cook, until heated all around—should be about 5 minutes.

The hash is ready, wait until it cools, and store it in the fridge. When you want to breakfast, you just have to reheat the hash and prepare the eggs like so:

1. Place hash in a skillet, and reheat over medium heat. Sautéing for 5 to 7 minutes. Move to the eggs. Melt the remaining tablespoon of butter in a skillet over medium heat. Add 2 eggs. Fry on one side until the edges are golden and the white is set.

2. It's time to plate. Place a cup of cauliflower hash on a plate, and top with one egg.

Recipe #18 – Keto Pinwheels

I used to eat a lot of tortillas—they're so crispy and crunchy. But, as many Keto dieters have found: they're not as low-carb as they *should* for our diet.

Substituting tortillas for meat is not something new, but it doesn't stop these pinwheels from being delicious:

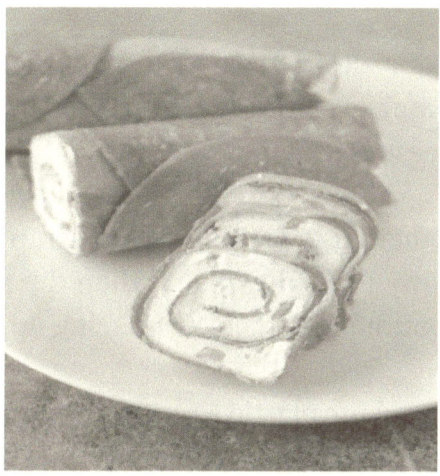

They will be the much needed lighter relief, after guzzling so much chicken and bacon goodness. These can last a lot of time in the freezer, and they're perfect for a snack or a side-dish.

Ingredients

- 8 oz. Block of cream cheese
- 8 to 10 thin slices of pepperoni
- 8 to 10 thin slices of Genoa salami
- 4 tablespoons of finely diced Dill pickles

Preparation

I keep it simple with just pickles, but feel free to go wild on your meals as you see fit! Just make sure it's all Keto-friendly.

1. Get the cream cheese block out of the fridge, and let it drop to room temperature. Whip until fluffy. Spread a large piece of plastic wrap, and then spread the cream cheese in a 1/4-inch thick rectangle in the center.

2. Spread your desired garnish over the cream cheese. Layer salami over the cream cheese. Overlap until all cream cheese is covered.

3. Place another large piece of plastic wrap over the salami layer. Gently press down, and then flip the rectangle so that the bottom cheese layer is facing up.

4. Carefully peel the plastic wrap off the cream cheese layer. Roll into a log shape, removing the bottom layer of plastic wrap slowly as you turn.

5. With the pinwheel done, place it in a tight plastic wrap. Refrigerate for about 4 hours minimum—preferably overnight. Slice into preferred thickness before eating.

Recipe #19 – Keto Salad Dressing

A nutritious dressing made with healthy fats and full of flavor—it can last a lot of time in the fridge as well!

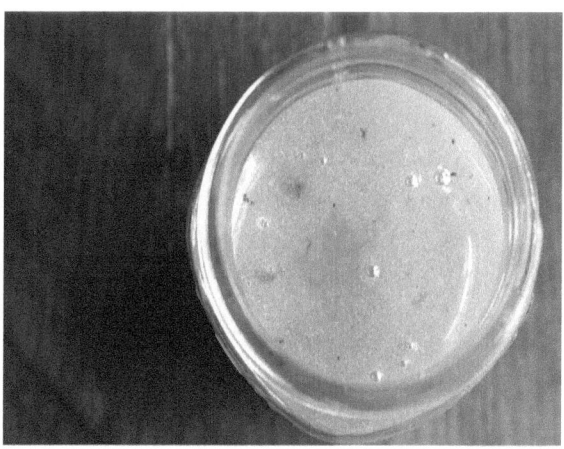

This recipe yields almost an entire cup of dressing. Just drizzle it over your greens and other vegetables to make those salads extra tasty!

Ingredients

- 1/4 Cup of mayonnaise
- 1 Tablespoon of Dijon mustard
- 1/4 Cup of extra virgin olive oil (alternatively, avocado oil)
- 2 Tablespoons of MCT oil
- 2 Garlic cloves
- 2 Tablespoons of fresh lemon juice
- 2 Tablespoons of freshly chopped herbs, your preference (parsley, basil, oregano, etc.)

- Salt and pepper to taste

Preparation

1. Peel and crush the garlic. Add garlic, mayo, lemon juice, mustard, and oils in the jar, and season to taste with salt and pepper.

2. Add the herbs (basil is always a nice touch!). Cover the jar with a lid and shake well. Store in fridge, up to a whole week! Be sure to shake well before drizzling your salads.

Recipe #20 – Keto Shrimps

I'm not an avid fan of seafood myself, but it does the body well, and in the case of shrimps, they're Keto-friendly!

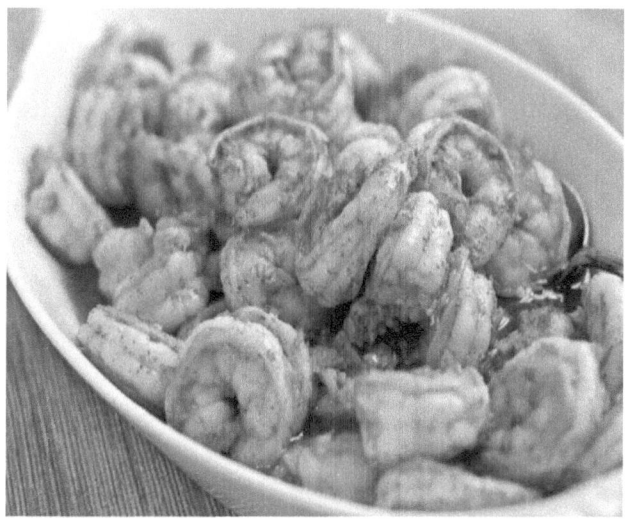

Whether you go crazy for shrimps, or feel like you have to provide your body with a balanced diet, you will enjoy these shrimps—they're tasty, and they're excellent for meal prep!

Ingredients

- 40 medium shrimp, peeled and deveined
- 2 Tablespoons of olive (or avocado) oil
- 2 Garlic cloves, minced
- 1 Teaspoon of ground cumin
- 1 Teaspoon of chili powder
- 1/2 Teaspoon of onion powder
- 1/2 Teaspoon of salt

Preparation

1. Whisk together 1 tablespoon of olive (or avocado) oil, garlic, cumin, chili, onion powder, and salt in a medium bowl.

2. Add in the shrimp, and toss to fully coat. Cover and refrigerate for at least 10 minutes, up to 24 hours. Heat a large cast iron skillet, on high, for 2 minutes.

3. Add remaining olive (or avocado) oil and shrimp. Cook shrimp in the skillet, on medium-high heat until pink—about 5 minutes.

You can freeze and store them safely in the freezer. Reheat in microwave or frying pan, and serve along with a tasty green salad and cubed cheese!

Recipe #21 – Keto Thai Turkey Wrap

This meal is perfect for meal prep, and you can have it as dinner or lunch—Just get your crunchy greens out, serve the turkey, and enjoy!

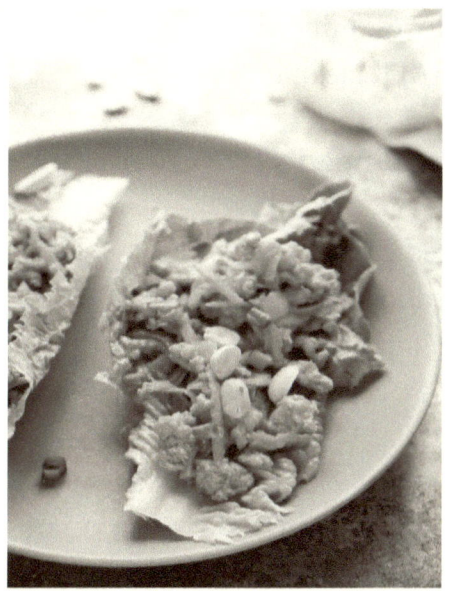

Ingredients

For the sauce, you will need

- 1/4 Cup of peanut butter
- 3 Tablespoons of soy sauce
- 2 Tablespoons of rice vinegar
- 2 Tablespoons of water
- 1 Tablespoon of lime juice
- 1 Teaspoon of Sesame oil

For the filling, you will need

- 1 Tablespoon of olive oil (alternatively, avocado oil)
- 1 Tablespoon of Thai red curry paste
- 1/4 Onion, finely chopped
- 1/2 Green peppers, finely chopped
- 3 garlic cloves, minced
- 1 1/2 – 1 1/4 lb. lean ground turkey

To serve, you will need

- Your stored greens
- Your shredded cheddar cheese
- 1/2 Green onions

Preparation

1. Add all the sauce ingredients in a jar, seal, and shake until well combined.

2. Add olive (or avocado) oil to a pan, and let it heat. Once hot, add in the garlic, onions, and red curry paste—Be sure to stir evenly so that the red curry paste is thoroughly heated and mixed with the onions and garlic. Should be around 2 to 3 minutes.

3. Add the ground turkey, break the chunks with a spatula, and cook for about 5 to 7 minutes. Make sure the turkey is cooked through, no pink should remain. Add the sauce evenly over the ground turkey, stir to combine. Remove from the heat.

To serve

1. Spoon 1/4 Cup of the ground turkey into a leaf of your greens. Sprinkle with the green onions and shedder cheese.

Storing it in the fridge is simple—Allow the turkey mixture to cool, portion it out into 1/2 – 3/4 cup portions and store in the fridge. Up to 4 days.

You can store the remaining portions for the other 3 days in the freezer just as well.

In both cases, you just reheat until steaming hot in the microwave.

Recipe #22 – Keto Meat Eggs & Veggies Breakfast

Scrambled eggs, the usual suspect of many Keto dishes, accompanied with hearty veggies and meat. Nutritious, delicious, easy to prepare, and easier to store.

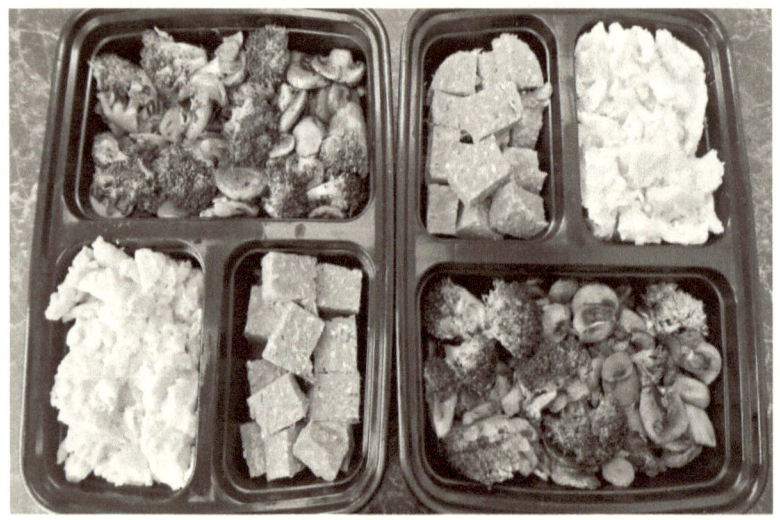

Making your own breakfast can't get any faster than this!

Ingredients

- 7 Eggs
- 2 Tablespoon of butter
- Salt and pepper to taste
- Meat of your choosing: sausages, bacon, salami, etc.

Preparation

For the eggs

1. Crack and mix the eggs in a bowl, add a tablespoon of butter to a heated pan, and add the eggs. Let the eggs set on the bottom, and stir gently—about 3 to 4 times. Bring the eggs from the bottom to the top.

2. Once they've set to the bottom again, fold the eggs over to ensure the mixture cooks. Add salt and pepper to taste. Remove from pan, allow to cool, and pop into your containers.

For the vegetables

1. Add the remaining tablespoon of butter to a frying pan, heat, and cook your vegetables of choice until they've softened. I personally cook broccoli and mushrooms, but there is a lot you can pick.

2. Remove from pan, allow to cool, and pop into your containers.

For the meat

1. You can go for sausages, bacon, and even salami, the sky is the limit here! You can have your meats whole, or you can chop into tinnier bits. Either way, store into containers.

2. Fry up your meat before heating. Reheat your foods briefly for a few minutes in a microwave while you fry

your meat and there you have it—filling Keto breakfast in just minutes!

Recipe #23 – Keto Caramelized Chips

Salty. Crispy. Coconut flavored. Keto-friendly. These chips are delicious as a snack or even as a salad garnish!

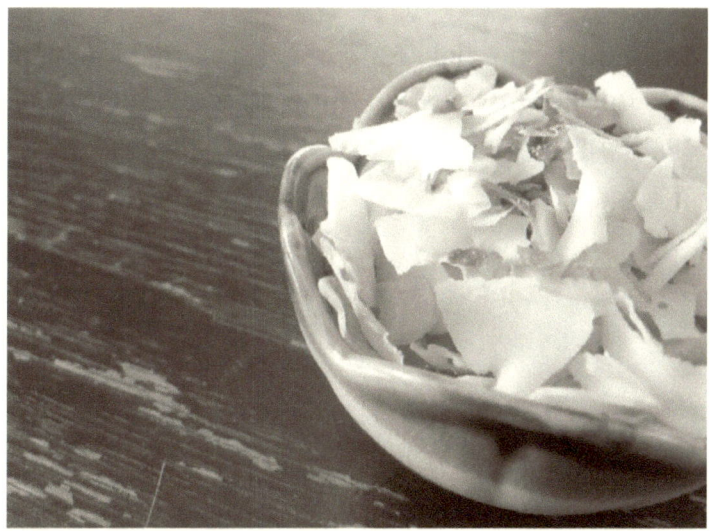

You can get them done in no time and they're pretty cheap too!

Ingredients

- 1 Cup of sweetened coconut chips
- 1/4 Cup of salt
- A pinch of cinnamon

Preparation

1. Add salt and cinnamon to a small bowl and mix well. Set aside.

2. Heat a pan, medium heat, for about 2 minutes. Add the coconut flakes, distributing them evenly to form a shallow layer in the bottom of the pan—Be sure to stir frequently, as they begin to crisp quickly. Once the flakes are toasty enough, remove from pan.

3. Sprinkle the hot flakes into the salt-cinnamon blend, and toss until evenly coated. Allow to cool, and then store in an air-tight container.

Conclusion

Whew, it has been a long trek from the introduction.

First, we went over the details of the Ketogenic diet, learned how does it all work, and how you can make it work for *you*.

Then, we switched over to the wonders of meal prep, how much time it can save you, and how efficient will it make your life and specially your diet!

We entered into proper Keto meal prep, reviewed several proposed weeks' worth of Keto meal prep, and gave you instructions and alternatives for your meals—Don't forget that this is not a strict diet plan, but rather a suggested plan with enough leeway to use your creativity.

Finally, we browsed a multitude of Keto-friendly recipes with many different ingredients and options. Most of the dishes here don't need any fancy hard-to-get ingredients. In fact, odds are you can prepare many of these without having to go out of your house, as you probably have some of the required ingredients laying around.

With this information in your head, tools in your kitchen, and ingredients in your fridge, you're *totally* poised to start an efficient Keto diet.

Whenever you want a refresher, or just a good look at the process of Ketosis to better fine tune your nutrient intake, you can open this book and refer to any part.

Dieting is not rocket science by any means, but as all controlled practices, it requires practice and tuning. Don't be afraid of trying new things, or experimenting with your own ideas!

You don't have to follow *my* footsteps, nor the footsteps of others, you just have to seek what I sought, and you'll eventually come around your own path.

Final Words

I would like to thank you for purchasing my book and I hope I have been able to help you and educate you on something new.

If you have enjoyed this book and would like to share your positive thoughts, could you please take 30 seconds of your time to go back and give me a review on my Amazon book page.

I greatly appreciate seeing these reviews because it helps me share my hard work.

You can leave me a review on Amazon.com.

Again, thank you and I wish you all the best!

www.ingramcontent.com/pod-product-compliance
Lightning Source LLC
Chambersburg PA
CBHW031125080526
44587CB00011B/1116